The Ketogenic Diet:

The Ultimate Guide to a Healthy Keto Diet

J. CEESAY

Legal & Disclaimer

The information contained in this book and its contents is not designed to replace or take the place of any form of medical or professional advice; and is not meant to replace the need for independent medical, financial, legal or other professional advice or services, as may be required. The content and information in this book has been provided for educational and entertainment purposes only.

The content and information contained in this book has been compiled from sources deemed reliable, and it is accurate to the best of the Author's knowledge, information and belief. However, the Author cannot guarantee its accuracy and validity and cannot be held liable for any errors and/or omissions. Further, changes are periodically made to this book as and when needed. Where appropriate and/or necessary, you must consult a professional (including but not limited to your doctor, attorney, financial advisor or such other professional advisor) before using any of the suggested remedies, techniques, or information in this book.

Upon using the contents and information contained in this book, you agree to hold harmless the Author from and against any damages, costs, and expenses, including any legal fees potentially resulting from the application of any of the information provided by this book. This disclaimer applies to any loss, damages or injury caused by the use and application, whether directly or indirectly, of any advice or information presented, whether for breach of contract, tort, negligence, personal injury, criminal intent, or under any other cause of action.

You agree to accept all risks of using the information presented inside this book.

You agree that by continuing to read this book, where appropriate and/or necessary, you shall consult a professional (including but not limited to your doctor, attorney, or financial advisor or such other advisor as needed) before using any of the suggested remedies, techniques, or information in this book.

Table of Contents

Vanilla Cream Delight

Conclusion

Introduction

This book is intended to be a starter guide about the Keto Diet to help you get started quickly with the basics. It is not intended to be a replacement for a scientific or a detailed research paper or book about the Ketogenic Diet or low carbohydrate diets and does not pretend to be.

After learning about the Keto Diet, only the best of health awaits you, and success in overcoming diabetes, hypertension, and obesity is not beyond your reach. You'll see that controlling your carbohydrate intake is the smartest and easiest way to lose weight and diet with less effort than thought possible.

Countless others and I are a true testament to its success in weight loss and healthy living. Many people all over the world are successfully taking back their health with the Keto Diet.

As part of the Keto Diet, you will need to significantly reduce the amount of carbohydrates you consume and focus more on consuming healthy fats. Although this is a high fat and low carb diet, don't be alarmed until you read further about the Keto Diet.

For background purposes, American adult males and females consume almost 50 percent of their daily calories from carbohydrates. In a standard Ketogenic Diet, on average approximately 70 percent of calories come from fat, about 25 percent comes from protein, and about five (5) percent comes from carbohydrates. These percentages could vary in range somewhat depending on the individual and their specific circumstances.

Fat, protein and carbohydrates are called Macronutrients (often referred to as "macros") which are required in large amounts in the human diet so that your body can grow, develop and repair itself. These macronutrients provide energy for your body in the form of calories.

These are average values for the caloric values per gram of each Macronutrient.

- 9 calories per gram of fat
- 4 calories per gram of protein
- 4 calories per gram of carbohydrates

In concert with Macronutrients, your body works with and needs essential Micronutrients which are very tiny amounts of vitamins and minerals to help your body maintain the proper energy levels, normal metabolism, good cell function, and to feel good both mentally and physically. As a part of Micronutrients, you may have heard of *Macro Minerals* (required in larger amounts) versus *Trace Minerals* (required in very tiny amounts).

- *Macro Minerals* - the top macro minerals your body needs are magnesium, sulfur and multiple electrolytes consisting of calcium, chloride, phosphorous, potassium, and sodium.

- *Trace Minerals* - the top trace minerals you need are chromium, copper, iodine, iron, manganese, molybdenum, selenium, and zinc.

You might be wondering and saying, "but what about protein?" Will I get enough? No worries. This diet also encourages you to consume adequate and moderate protein.

However, you can't eat too much protein to get the best results. Otherwise it may raise your insulin level high enough to prevent weight loss. While protein does not raise your insulin level as high as carbohydrates, it still does. Fat has a minimal and the least effect in your insulin levels. Many do not realize this.

The ketogenic diet is a great option for most people and is shown to be highly effective. However, if you are suffering from certain diseases or ailments, it is advised that you consult your doctor first. Making dietary changes can affect your treatment and body as well. If they say it is okay, then go ahead with it. The diet is effective if you follow it properly and consistently for some time. It won't show results in a day or two but will have long-lasting effects that you will benefit from.

Ketogenic diets are not to be taken as mere diets but an embedded part of your new lifestyle. The effectiveness and success of ketogenic diets will be felt, experienced, and seen only when you find the discipline and courage to take the first step forward.

As you can see, ketogenic diets can help you get a lot of benefits, and it is those benefits which will keep you going when you take up this change in diet. Imagine being able to see the scales report back your loss of weight within a few weeks of being in ketosis and being able to keep it there in the optimal range without fear of rebound. How about visiting your cardiologist after a sustained drive in ketosis and having him take you off medications for high blood pressure and other metabolic issues? These are not far-fetched notions and can be achieved with commitment.

A good ketogenic diet will help you get your energy from fats, a more sustainable energy source than carbohydrates.

Chapter 1: Benefits of the Keto Diet

Recent research has found that the Keto Diet may be associated with some improvements in some cardiovascular risk factors, such as obesity, type 2 diabetes and HDL cholesterol levels although long-term research is not currently available.

Regulates Your Appetite

Most often the reason why I have ended up giving up on a diet plan is because I would feel so tired but mostly hungry. Most diets that I have attempted to follow in the past were so restrictive that I hardly had the satisfaction of eating enough and feeling full.

The Keto diet won't make you feel famished beyond the first few days when your body is still getting used to fat as the source of its energy. When your body starts burning the fat stored, you will feel energized and the high fat content makes you feel full.

It doesn't feel like you are actually dieting because you still get to eat most of the things that you love except maybe your carbs. Unlike carbs, fat doesn't get digested quickly so you feel full longer.

Therefore, you won't feel hungry so often. When you consume more carbs, especially high glycemic carbs, your body burns them off quickly and you end up feeling hungry soon enough. By implementing this diet, you are actually taking care of these random hunger pains and regulating your appetite with fat and high-fiber, low glycemic vegetables.

Regulating your appetite also plays an important role in helping you lose weight. When you don't feel hungry often you will end up eating less than before and reducing the number of calories you consume. Therefore, you only have to worry about an increased number of calories to burn.

Helps in Managing Your Blood Sugar Levels

We have already seen how the intake of carbs is responsible for the release of glucose into your bloodstream. This is the reason why we immediately experience a surge in our energy levels when we consume carbs.

As you know, the hormone called *insulin* is responsible for regulating our blood sugar levels. However, insulin doesn't function as it is supposed to for certain people. It doesn't regulate the blood sugar levels which ultimately results in *Type 2 diabetes*.

This phenomenon of insulin not functioning properly over a long period of time **is known as "insulin resistance"**. Recent research has shown that Insulin resistance is a primary cause for cardiovascular disease risk.

Therefore, if you are insulin resistant, the Keto Diet can help you alleviate the risk of type 2 diabetes. This is because the amount of sugar released into your bloodstream is reduced as a result of reduced intake of carbs. Even if your insulin doesn't function the way it is intended to, your blood sugar levels won't increase, and you probably don't have to worry about Type-2 diabetes.

The Keto Diet is suitable even if you are suffering from Type 2 diabetes. It can actually help you manage your diabetes with minimal medication thanks to the reduced production of sugar/glucose.

Helps in Regulating Your Blood Pressure Levels

Hypertension has become a common household problem these days. This is responsible for increasing your risk factors for various disorders related to the kidneys, cardiac disorders, etc. Therefore, you simply cannot afford to turn a blind eye to hypertension.

One of the common suggestions prescribed by physicians, as part of treating hypertension, is to reduce your intake of salt. This is because salt is capable of increasing your blood pressure levels.

Well, not all of us can take this suggestion with a pinch of salt, can we? Your meals won't taste the same without adding salt to them.

Here is the good news – you don't have to cut back on your salt intake as long as it is not excessive if you are following this diet.

The Keto Diet helps in managing your blood pressure levels even without reducing your intake of salt. Let's look at how this diet is capable of doing this:

• *When you are consuming foods which are rich in carbs, your blood sugar levels will automatically increase.* When there is a surge in your blood sugar levels and if you are insulin resistant, it ends up constricting your blood vessels. The constriction in the blood vessels has an impact on your blood pressure levels and causes it to increase.

• *By reducing your carb intake, you are essentially managing your blood sugar levels.* When your blood sugar is under control, you don't have to worry about constricted blood vessels or hypertension unless you have a specific underlying condition that is causing the hypertension.

- *An important reason behind hypertension is insulin resistance.* We just saw how the Keto Diet plays an important role in managing your insulin resistance by making you reduce your intake of carbs.

- You will see in a bit how the Keto Diet helps to reduce the amount of visceral fat stored in our bodies. *The reduction in the amount of visceral fat helps in managing your insulin resistance*. This also helps to lower your risk when it comes to several cardiac disorders. With insulin resistance managed, you are reducing one more risk factor for hypertension.

- You already know that the Keto Diet encourages the body to burn the fat stored in your body. *As part of burning the fat, the sodium and potassium content in your kidneys get flushed out*.

- This results in an electrolyte imbalance, which can be addressed by the increased intake of salt and bone broth, beef broth and chicken broth. *As you can see, you are actually managing your hypertension with this diet, without reducing your intake of salt.*

Helps to Get Rid of Visceral Fat

When your body digests the foods that you consume, the fat present gets deposited in different parts of your body, but you have no control over where it goes. Depending on the places where your fat gets deposited, the associated risk factors will vary. The fat that we consume gets stored under our skin (**subcutaneous fat)** or gets deposited in the abdominal cavity (**visceral fat).**

It is also capable of affecting the manner in which the different organs in your body function due to the crowding of your organs due to the visceral fat.

When there is an increase in the amount of visceral fat deposited in your body, it causes inflammation of organs. Insulin resistance and also impairs your body's metabolism. **When the metabolism of your body is impacted, your efforts to lose weight will also be impacted**. In fact, it will take you longer than usual to lose weight. Therefore, you have to make sure that your visceral fat deposits are under control.

The Keto Diet is capable of reducing the visceral fat stored in our bodies. This stubborn fat is digested by the body to derive energy. By getting rid of excess visceral fat, you are actually reducing your risk factors for various health disorders. Your efforts to lose weight will also not be compromised by the presence of visceral fat.

Chapter 2: Ketogenic Diet: Food List

Foods to Eat

Following are the foods that are emphasized on a keto diet.

- Healthy, fatty fish such as tuna, salmon, etc.

- Healthy oils such as avocado oil, coconut oil, olive oil, etc.

- All types of full-fat cheese and full-fat cream cheese, sour cream, crème Fraiche.

- Unsweetened almond/coconut milk, or another nut milk

- Eggs

- Butter, total fat

- Avocados

- Walnuts, almonds, cashews, and other nuts

- Chia seed and flax seed

- Olives

- Bacon

- Unsweetened beverages

- Heavy cream

- Healthy low carb, non-starchy veggies such as leek, fennel, spinach, kale, broccoli, tomatoes, other greens, etc.

- All types of berries but in small quantities

- Herbs and most spices

Foods to Avoid

- All types of sweetened beverages, fruit juices, and other sweetened drinks.

- All types of starchy vegetables including white potatoes, sweet potatoes, etc.

- Commercial fried foods, snacks, and bakery products including sugar-based desserts.

- Wheat pasta, bread, rice, cereals, and other high carb wheat products.

- All types of commercial processed food items.

- Legumes and beans

- Fruits can be consumed but a small quantity

- Alcohol and unhealthy cooking oils

Chapter 3: Breakfast Recipes

Breakfast Mexican Omelet

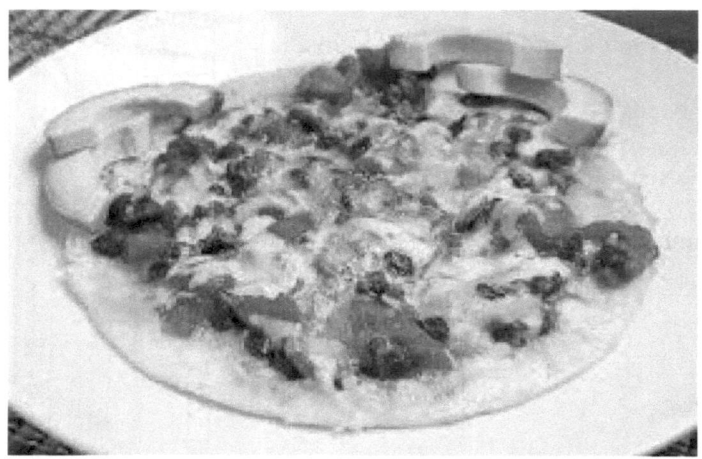

Prep time: 4 minutes

Cook time: 9 minutes

Number of Servings: 1

Ingredients

- ½ tablespoon lime juice

- 2 eggs

- 1 tablespoon water

- 1 tablespoon crumbled bacon

- 1/2 tablespoon butter

- ¼ avocado

- ½ cup hand-shredded Mexican cheese

- 2 tablespoon Pace Thick and Chunky Medium Salsa

Directions

1. Melt the butter in a microwaveable bowl in the microwave.

2. Quickly whip the wet ingredients in a microwaveable bowl, can be the same bowl as before.

3. Microwave for one minute.

4. Place on warm plate.

5. Top with all the rest of the ingredients.

6. Combine the wet ingredients in a zip-lock bag, except the butter and water. Refrigerate. Combine the water and butter in a zip-lock bag.

Nutritional Value:

Calories: 275,

Total Fat: 21,

Protein: 17g,

Total Carbs: 3.2g,

Dietary Fiber: 2g,

Sugar: 2g,

Sodium: 230mg

Breakfast Casserole

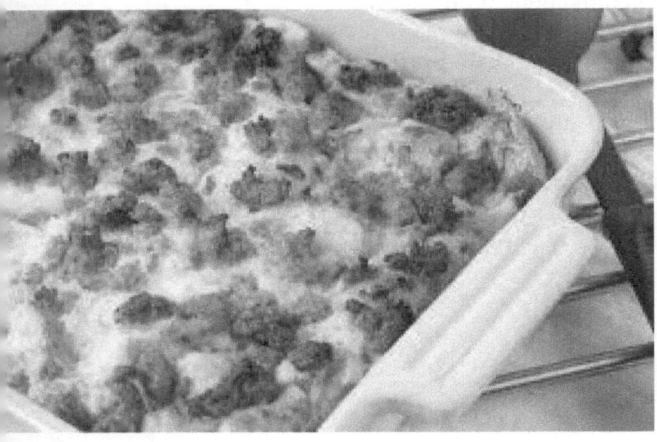

Prep time: 4 minutes

Cook time: 19 minutes

Number of Servings: 4

Ingredients

- 8 oz Sausage, Cooked and Crumbled
- 1 cup hot salsa
- 4 eggs
- 2 chopped green onions
- ¼ cup hand-shredded pepper jack or cheddar cheese
- ½ bell pepper, chopped, your choice of color

Directions

1. Place oven rack to the middle shelf setting.
2. Heat oven to 400 degrees.
3. Cook the peppers until soft.
4. Spray or grease the baking dishes excessively. Eggs stick when baked.
5. Layer ingredients in 4 individual baking dishes, like Corning ware "grab-its," any bakeware that holds one cup servings.
6. Layer with sausage first, then peppers, then cheese.
7. Add one whipped egg to each baking dish. Sprinkle with green onions.
8. Bake for 18 minutes, until eggs are set.
9. Place cooled casseroles in individual freezer bags. Reheat in microwave for 2-3 minutes until hot.

Nutritional Value:

Calories: 195,

Total Fat: 11g,

Protein: 19g,

Total Carbs: 3g,

Dietary Fiber: 1g,

Sugar: 0,

Sodium: 112mg

Cinnamon Chocolate Smoothie

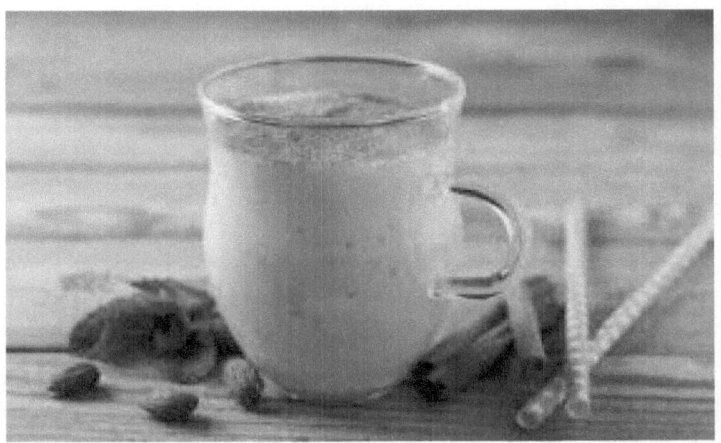

Prep time: 4 minutes

Cook time: 0 minutes

Number of Servings: 1

Ingredients

- ½ cup firm Tofu

- 2 tablespoon cocoa powder

- 1 scoop chocolate protein powder

- 2 tablespoon cinnamon

- 2 sweetener packets

- 1 cup almond milk, unsweetened

- 4 ice cubes

Directions

1. Place all the ingredients in a blender, pulse until desired consistency, and serve.

2. Refrigerate the tofu. Place all the dry ingredients into one snack sized zip-lock bag.

Nutritional Value:

Calories: 273,

Total Fat: 15g,

Protein: 33g,

Total Carbs: 9g,

Dietary Fiber: 20g,

Sugar: 2g,

Sodium: 214mg

Avocado Egg Muffins

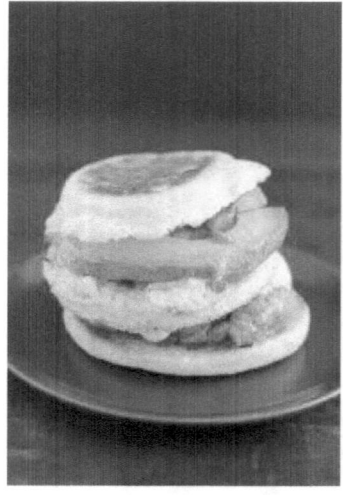

Prep Time: 8-10 min.

Cooking Time: 12 min.

Number of Servings: 4

Ingredients:

- 1 ½ cups coconut milk
- 2 avocados, diced
- 4 ½ ounces (grated or shredded) cheese
- ½ cup almond flour
- 5 bacon slices, cooked and crumbled
- 5 eggs, beaten
- 2 tablespoon butter
- 3 spring onions, diced
- 1 teaspoon oregano
- ¼ cup flaxseed meal
- 1 ½ tablespoon lemon juice
- 1 teaspoon minced garlic
- 1 teaspoon onion powder
- 1 teaspoon salt
- Pinch of pepper
- 1 teaspoon baking powder
- 1 ½ cups water

Directions:

1. Whisk together the wet ingredients.
2. Gradually stir in the dry ingredients; mix until turns smooth. Stir in the avocado, bacon, onions, and cheese.
3. Add the mixture into 16 muffin cups.
4. Arrange Instant Pot over a dry platform in your kitchen. Open its top lid and switch it on.
5. In the pot, pour water. Arrange a trivet or steamer basket inside that came with Instant Pot. Now place/arrange the 8 cups over the trivet/basket.
6. Close top lid to create a locked chamber; make sure that safety valve is in locking position.
7. Find and press "MANUAL" cooking function; timer to 12 minutes with default "HIGH" pressure mode.
8. Allow the pressure to build to cook the ingredients.
9. After cooking time is over, press "CANCEL" setting. Find and press "QPR" cooking function. This setting is for quick release of inside pressure.
10. Slowly open the lid, take out the cooked recipe in serving plates or serving bowls and enjoy the keto recipe.
11. Repeat the same process.

Nutritional Values (Per Serving):

Calories - 146

Fat – 11g

Saturated Fat – 3g

Trans Fat – 0g

Carbohydrates – 4g

Fiber – 2g

Sodium – 356mg

Protein – 6g

Chapter 4: Main Dishes

Chicken Lettuce Wraps

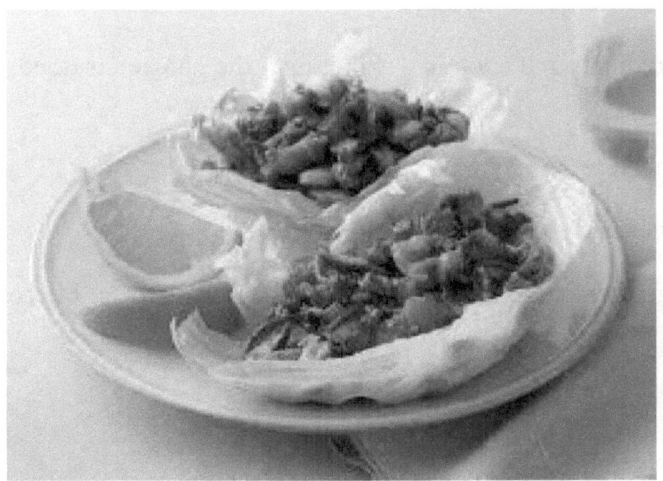

Prep time: 10minutes

Cook time: 10minutes

Number of Servings: 1

Ingredients

- 1 chicken breast, boneless, diced into 1-inch size pieces

- 1 cup diced or sliced fresh mushrooms

- ½ cup diced water chestnuts (from a can, drained)

- 1 tablespoon olive oil

- 1 tablespoon onion, minced

- 1 tablespoon minced garlic

- 1 tablespoon teriyaki sauce

- garlic powder, only a dash

- onion powder, just a dash

- oregano, one dash

- cayenne pepper, a small dash

- salt /pepper

Directions

1. Mix the ingredients and cook in a skillet until the chicken is done, about 10 minutes.

2. Shred the chicken

3. Place in leaves and roll

4. Place all ingredients into one freezer bag except the lettuce. Microwave one minute and serve.

Nutritional Value:

Calories: 145,

Total Fat: 1g,

Protein: 35g,

Dietary Fiber: 1g,

Total Carbs: 4g,

Sugar: 0g,

Sodium: 100mg

Indian Chicken Curry

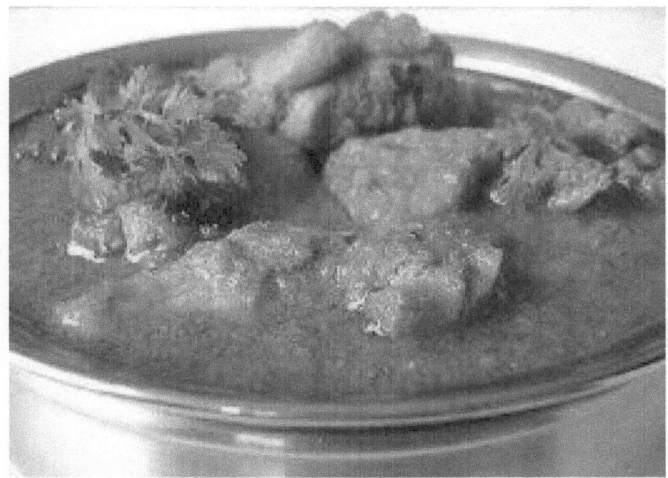

Prep Time: 2 Hours

Number of Servings: 4

Ingredients:

- 6 chicken thighs, cut into small pieces

- 1 onion, diced

- 4 cloves of garlic, minced

- 1 tablespoon of salt

- 2 tablespoon of red curry paste

- 2 tablespoons of curry, powdered

- 2 tablespoon of soy sauce

- 5 drops of Stevia

- 3 tablespoons of cilantro, fresh, chopped and extra for garnish

- ¼ cup of extra virgin olive oil

- 3 tablespoon of coconut oil

- ½ cup of heavy cream

- 2 tablespoons of cornstarch

- 2 tablespoons of cold water

- 1 lime, fresh and juice only

Directions:

1. Use a large bowl and add in the chicken thigh pieces, onion, garlic, dash of salt, red curry paste, powdered curry, soy sauce, stevia, cilantro and extra virgin olive oil. Stir well to mix.

2. Cover the bowl and set into the fridge to marinate for 1 hour.

3. After this time place a large skillet over medium to high heat. Add in the coconut oil and once the oil is hot enough add in the marinated chicken. Cook for 8 to 10 minutes or until the chicken is cooked through.

4. Pour in the coconut milk and bring the mixture to a boil. Once boiling reduce the heat to low. Cover and cook for 30 to 40 minutes. Make sure to stir the chicken every 5 to 10 minutes.

5. Add in the heavy cream after this time and increase the heat to high. Bring the mixture to a boil.

6. While the mixture is coming to a boil add the cornstarch and water into a small bowl. Whisk to make a slurry and pour into the chicken mixture. Stir well to mix and cook for 5 minutes or until thick in consistency.

7. Add in the fresh lime juice and a dash of salt.

8. Remove from heat and serve.

Nutritional Value:

Calories: 408,

Fat: 32 grams,

Carbs: 7 grams,

Protein: 23 grams

No Bake Cheesecake

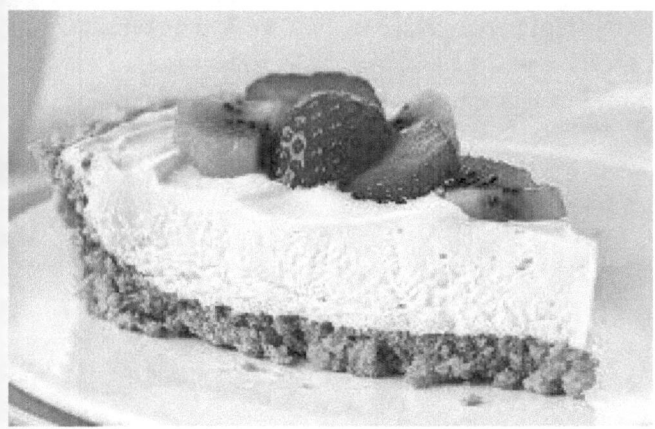

Prep Time: 6 Hours and 15 Minutes

Number of Servings: 4

Ingredients:

- ½ cup of almond flour
- ¼ cup of butter, melted
- 16 ounces of cream cheese, soft
- ¾ cup of artificial sweetener
- ½ tablespoon of pure vanilla
- ½ tablespoon of lemon juice, fresh
- ½ tablespoon of salt

Directions:

1. Spray a muffin pan with cooking spray and line with paper muffin lines.

2. Use a large bowl and add in the almond flour and butter. Stir well until mixed. Pour this mixture into the bottom of each muffin cup. Press flat to make a crust.

3. Use a separate bowl and add in the cream cheese, artificial sweetener, pure vanilla, fresh lemon juice and dash of salt. Beat with an electric mixer until creamy in consistency. Pour this mixture over the crusts.

4. Place the muffin pan into the freezer to freeze for 2 hours.

5. Remove after this time and transfer into the fridge to thaw for 3 to 4 hours. Serve. Flank Steak Stuffed with Pancetta and Goat Cheese This is a great tasting keto friendly dish you can make for lunch or dinner.

Nutritional Value:

Calories: 195,

Fat: 19 grams,

Carbs: 3 grams,

Protein: 3 grams

Italian Eggplant Lasagna

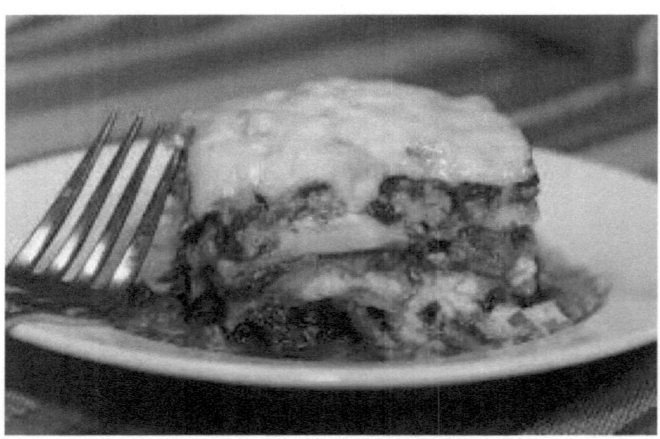

Prep time: 1 Hour and 45 Minutes

Number of Servings: 4

Ingredients:

- 1 eggplant, sliced thinly

- 2 tablespoons of salt

- 6 tablespoon of extra virgin olive oil

- 1 pound of Italian sausage

- 2 cups of ricotta cheese

- 2 cups of marinara sauce

- 3 cups of mozzarella cheese, shredded

- 2 cups of Parmesan cheese, grated

Directions:

1. Place the eggplant slices on a flat surface. Season with a dash of salt and set aside to sit for 20 to 30 minutes.

2. Preheat the oven to 400 degrees.

3. Pat dry the paper towels with a sheet of paper towels.

4. Drizzle the olive oil over the eggplant slices and place onto a large baking sheet. Place into the oven to roast for 10 minutes.

5. While the eggplant slices are roasting place a large skillet over medium heat. Add in the Italian sausage and cook for 10 to 12 minutes or until cooked through. Remove and set aside.

6. Reduce the temperature in the oven to 375 degrees.

7. Then use a large bowl and add in the Italian sausage and ricotta cheese. Stir well to mix. Pour half a cup of this mixture into the bottom of a large greased baking dish. Lay down 1/3 of the eggplant slices into the baking dish. Repeat the layers. Top off with the marinara sauce, mozzarella cheese and Parmesan cheese.

8. Cover the baking dish with a sheet of aluminum foil. Place into the oven to bake for 30 to 40 minutes. Remove the aluminum foil and continue to bake for another 10 minutes or until browned.

9. Remove from the oven and allow cooling for 20 minutes before serving.

Nutritional Value:

Calories: 667,

Fat: 51 grams,

Carbs: 14 grams,

Protein: 38 grams

Steak Salad with Asian Spice

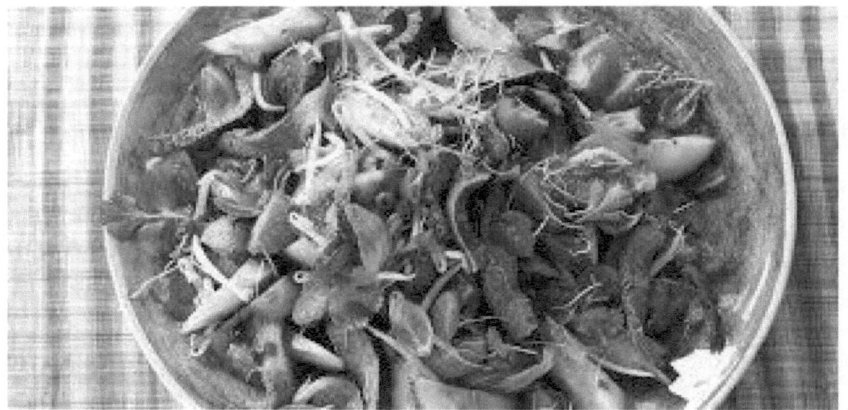

Prep time: 4 minutes

Cook time: 4 minutes

Number of Servings: 2

Ingredients

- 2 tablespoon sriracha sauce

- 1 tablespoon garlic, minced

- 1 tablespoon ginger, fresh, grated

- 1 bell pepper, yellow, cut into thin strips

- 1 bell pepper, red, cut into thin strips

- 1 tablespoon sesame oil, garlic

- 1 Splenda packet

- ½ tablespoon curry powder

- ½ tablespoon rice wine vinegar

- 8 oz. of beef sirloin, cut into strips

- 2 cups baby spinach, stemmed

- ½ head butter lettuce, torn or chopped into bite-sized pieces

Directions

1. Place the garlic, sriracha sauce, 1 tablespoon sesame oil, rice wine vinegar, and Splenda into a bowl and combine well.

2. Pour half of this mix into a zip-lock bag. Add the steak to marinade while you are preparing the salad.

3. Assemble the brightly colored salad by layering in two bowls.

4. Place the baby spinach into the bottom of the bowl. Place the butter lettuce next.

5. Mix the two peppers and place on top.

6. Remove the steak from the marinade and discard the liquid and bag.

7. Heat the sesame oil and quickly stir fry the steak until desired doneness, it should take about 3 minutes.

8. Place the steak on top of the salad.

9. Drizzle with the remaining dressing (other half of marinade mix).

10. Sprinkle sriracha sauce across the salad.

11. Combine the salad ingredients and place in a zip-lock bag in the fridge. Mix the marinade and halve into 2 zip-lock bags. Place the sriracha sauce into a small sealed container. Slice the steak and freeze in a zip-lock bag with the marinade. To prepare, mix the ingredients like the initial directions. Stir fry the marinated beef for 4 minutes to take into consideration the beef is frozen.

Nutritional Value:

Calories: 350,

Total Fat: 23g,

Protein: 28g,

Total Carbs: 7g,

Dietary Fiber: 3.5,

Sugar: 0,

Sodium: 267mg

Chicken Chow Mein Stir Fry

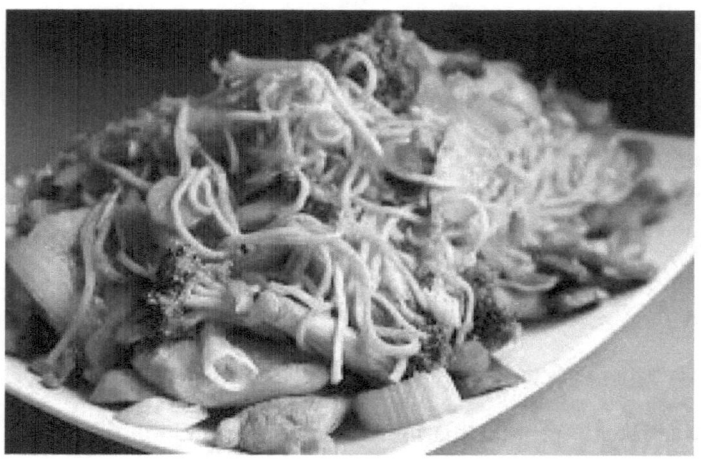

Prep time: 9 minutes

Cook time: 14 minutes

Number of Servings: 4

Ingredients

- 1/2 cup sliced onion

- 2 tablespoon Oil, sesame garlic flavored

- 4 cups shredded Bok-Choy

- 1 cup Sugar Snap Peas

- 1 cup fresh bean sprouts

- 3 stalks Celery, chopped

- 1 1/2 tablespoon minced Garlic

- 1 packet Splenda

- 1 cup Broth, chicken

- 2 tablespoon Soy Sauce

- 1 tablespoon ginger, freshly minced

- 1 tablespoon cornstarch

- 4 boneless Chicken Breasts, cooked/sliced thinly

Directions

1. Place the bok-choy, peas, celery in a skillet with 1 T garlic oil.

2. Stir fry until bok-choy is softened to liking.

3. Add remaining ingredients except for the cornstarch.

4. If too thin, stir cornstarch into ½ cup cold water. When smooth pour into skillet.

5. Bring cornstarch and chow mein to a one-minute boil. Turn off the heat source.

6. Stir sauce then for wait 4 minutes to serve, after the chow mein has thickened.

7. Freeze in covered containers. Heat for 2 minutes in the microwave before serving.

Nutritional Value:

Calories: 368,

Total Fat: 18g,

Protein: 42g,

Total Carbs: 12g,

Dietary Fiber: 16g,

Sugar: 6g,

Sodium: 746mg

Salmon with Bok-Choy

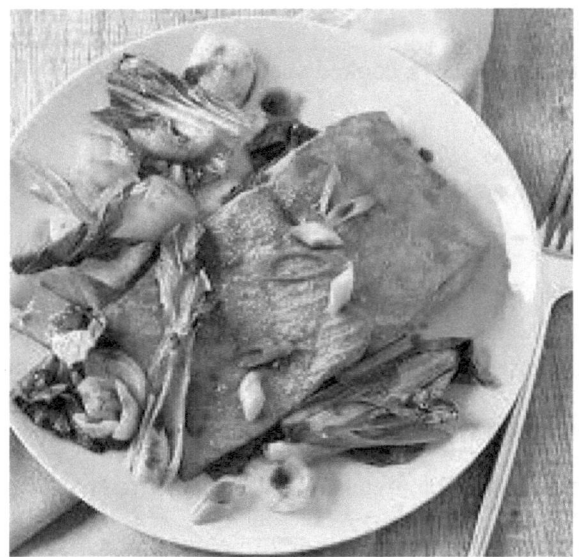

Prep time: 9 minutes

Cook time: 9 minutes

Number of Servings: 4

Ingredients

- 1 cup red peppers, roasted, drained
- 2 cups chopped bok-choy
- 1 tablespoon salted butter
- 5 oz. salmon steak
- 1 lemon, sliced very thinly
- ⅛ tablespoon black pepper
- 1 tablespoon olive oil
- 2 tablespoon sriracha sauce

Directions

1. Place oil in skillet

2. Place all but 4 slices of lemon in the skillet.

3. Sprinkle the bok choy with the black pepper.

4. Stir fry the bok-choy with the lemons.

5. Remove and place on four plates.

6. Place the butter in the skillet and stir fry the salmon, turning once.

7. Place the salmon on the bed of bok-choy.

8. Divide the red peppers and encircle the salmon.

9. Place a slice of lemon atop the salmon.

10. Drizzle with sriracha sauce.

11. Freeze the cooked salmon in individual zip-lock bags. Place the bok-choy, with the remaining ingredients into one cup containers. Microwave the salmon for one minute and the frozen bok choy for two. Assemble to serve.

Nutritional Value:

Calories: 410,

Total Fat: 30g,

Protein: 30g,

Total Carbs: 7g,

Dietary Fiber: 2g,

Sugar: 0g,

Sodium: 200mg

Chapter 5: Delicious Desserts

Almond Mug Cake

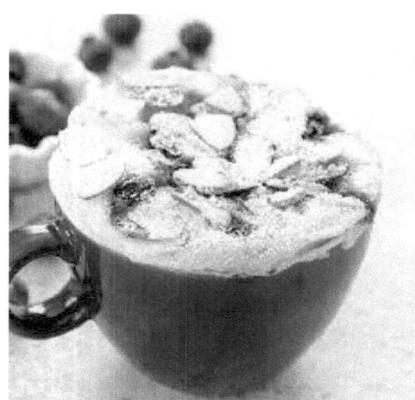

Prep Time: 8-10 min.

Cooking Time: 10 min.

Number of Servings: 1

Ingredients:

- 1/4 teaspoon baking powder
- 1/4 teaspoon vanilla extract
- 1 1/2 tablespoons cacao powder
- 1 egg, beaten
- 1/4 cup almond flour
- 1 teaspoon cinnamon powder
- 2 tablespoons stevia powder
- A pinch of salt

Directions:

1. Combine all ingredients in the bowl until well-combined. Add the mix in a heat-proof mug; cover with a foil.
2. Arrange Instant Pot over a dry platform in your kitchen. Open its top lid and switch it on.
3. In the pot, pour water. Arrange a trivet or steamer basket inside that came with Instant Pot. Now place/arrange the mug over the trivet/basket.
4. Close top lid to create a locked chamber; make sure that safety valve is in locking position.
5. Find and press "MANUAL" cooking function; timer to 10 minutes with default "HIGH" pressure mode.

6. Allow the pressure to build to cook the ingredients.
7. After cooking time is over, press "CANCEL" setting. Find and press "QPR" cooking function. This setting is for quick release of inside pressure.
8. Slowly open the lid, cool down the mug and serve warm.

Nutritional Values (Per Serving):

Calories - 138

Fat – 13g

Saturated Fat – 6g

Trans Fat – 0g

Carbohydrates – 7g

Fiber – 3g

Sodium – 73mg

Protein – 9g

Tapioca Keto Pudding

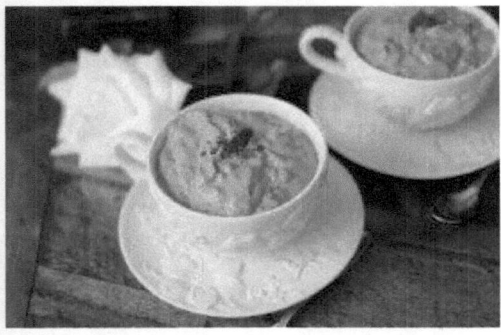

Prep Time: 8-10 min.

Cooking Time: 20 min.

Number of Servings: 4

Ingredients:

- 1 tablespoon Erythritol
- 1 teaspoon chia seeds
- 1 tablespoon tapioca
- 1 tablespoon butter
- 2 cup heavy cream
- 1/4 cup raspberries or strawberries, mashed

Directions:

1. Arrange Instant Pot over a dry platform in your kitchen. Open its top lid and switch it on.
2. Find and press "SAUTE" cooking function.
3. In the pot, add the cream; cook (while stirring) for 4-5 minutes.
4. Add the tapioca and stir it well. Add the Erythritol and butter.
5. In a bowl, mix the chia seeds and berries.
6. Add the berry mix in the pot and stir well.
7. Close top lid to create a locked chamber; make sure that safety valve is in locking position.
8. Find and press "MANUAL" cooking function; timer to 15 minutes with default "HIGH" pressure mode.
9. Allow the pressure to build to cook the ingredients.
10. After cooking time is over, press "CANCEL" setting. Find and press "QPR" cooking function. This setting is for quick release of inside pressure.
11. Add in serving bowls, cool down and place in the fridge for 2 hours.
12. Serve chilled.

Nutritional Values (Per Serving):

Calories - 246

Fat – 24g

Saturated Fat – 9g

Trans Fat – 0g

Carbohydrates – 10g

Fiber – 2g

Sodium – 183mg

Protein – 3g

Cream Chocolate Delight

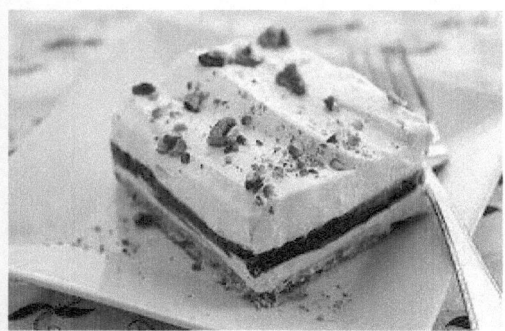

Prep Time: 8-10 min.

Cooking Time: 15 min.

Number of Servings: 4

Ingredients:

- 1 teaspoon orange zest
- 1 teaspoon stevia powder
- 2 heavy cream
- ¼ cup unsweetened dark chocolate, chopped
- 3 eggs
- 1 teaspoon vanilla extract
- ½ teaspoon salt

Directions:

1. Arrange Instant Pot over a dry platform in your kitchen. Open its top lid and switch it on.
2. Find and press "SAUTE" cooking function.
3. In the pot, add the heavy cream, chopped chocolate, stevia powder, vanilla extract, orange zest, and salt; cook (while stirring) until the chocolate is melted.
4. Crack eggs in the pot; stirring constantly. Remove from the instant pot. Add the mixture to 4 mason jars with loose lids.
5. In the pot, pour water. Arrange a trivet or steamer basket inside that came with Instant Pot. Now place/arrange the jars over the trivet/basket.
6. Close top lid to create a locked chamber; make sure that safety valve is in locking position.
7. Find and press "MANUAL" cooking function; timer to 10 minutes with default "HIGH" pressure mode.
8. Allow the pressure to build to cook the ingredients.

9. After cooking time is over, press "CANCEL" setting. Find and press "QPR" cooking function. This setting is for quick release of inside pressure.
10. Slowly open the lid, cool down the jars and chill in the fridge. Serve chilled.

Nutritional Values (Per Serving):

Calories - 254

Fat – 26g

Saturated Fat – 12g

Trans Fat – 0g

Carbohydrates – 5g

Fiber – 1g

Sodium – 168mg

Protein – 8g

Vanilla Cream Delight

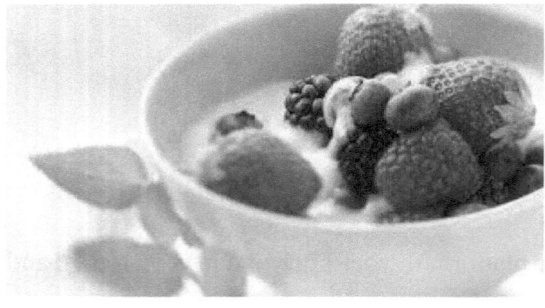

Prep Time: 8-10 min.

Cooking Time: 15 min.

Number of Servings: 4

Ingredients:

- 1 ½ cup heavy cream
- 1 teaspoon vanilla extract
- 8 large eggs
- ¾ cup unsweetened almond milk
- 1 vanilla bean
- 4 tablespoons stevia granular

Directions:

1. Cut the vanilla bean lengthwise using a knife and take out the seeds. Add in a mixing bowl.
2. Mix in the remaining ingredients. Whisk the mix thoroughly and add into 4 ramekins.
3. Arrange Instant Pot over a dry platform in your kitchen. Open its top lid and switch it on.
4. In the pot, pour 2 cups water. Arrange a trivet or steamer basket inside that came with Instant Pot. Now place/arrange the ramekins over the trivet/basket.
5. Close top lid to create a locked chamber; make sure that safety valve is in locking position.
6. Find and press "MANUAL" cooking function; timer to 15 minutes with default "HIGH" pressure mode.
7. Allow the pressure to build to cook the ingredients.
8. After cooking time is over, press "CANCEL" setting. Find and press "QPR" cooking function. This setting is for quick release of inside pressure.
9. Slowly open the lid, cool down the ramekins.
10. Chill in fridge and serve.

Nutritional Values (Per Serving):

Calories - 318

Fat – 26g

Saturated Fat – 7g

Trans Fat – 0g

Carbohydrates – 3g

Fiber – 0g

Sodium – 106mg

Protein – 13g

Conclusion

There you have it – the ketogenic diet. At this point, you already know what it is, why it's good for you, how to implement or introduce the ketogenic diet, how to tell if you've already reached a state of ketosis. You also have sample meal plans, tips for staying ketogenic while eating out, and delicious recipes to try at home. You know enough about the ketogenic diet to start enjoying its benefits.

The ketogenic diet is a great way to watch pounds melt away, quickly and safely. Your own body turns into a fat burning machine, using up stores of fat rather than glucose from the food you're eating for energy.

At the same time, it protects your heart and other muscles from damage since you're feeding them nourishing, healthy oils and lots of needed protein.

For the ketogenic diet to work, you don't need to count calories and weigh or measure your food necessarily, but as with all eating plans, you need to be honest with yourself about what you're eating and how much.

I want you to remember though, no matter how much you try to lose that extra body fat, you must take your age into consideration. Especially if you have already passed middle age, you need to accept that you can no longer have the body you had when you were 20 or 30. Sometimes, in the quest to be our best, we may forget that we have a wholesome, working body – far more than a lot of people can say.

But don't lose heart, while the time to look your "best" may have passed, the time to just shed a few pounds, enjoy your body and live a healthier life is now! Try your best to find a balance between living healthily and being happy with the body you have. Make sure to follow this simple cookbook guide to help you lose weight and live an overall healthier lifestyle. So, what are you waiting for – get slow cooking!

While virtually unlimited fats are allowed, it's good to get healthy, unsaturated fats that your body can easily digest and which won't clog your arteries; this means fats from fish, avocados, and peanuts, and olive oil. Lean protein choices are also better than fatty cuts of beef.

As with the rest of your food, you don't necessarily need to count carbohydrates, as long as you educate yourself about which foods are high in carbs and are sure to limit these in your diet.

If you do follow the ketogenic diet as recommended, you'll get a lean and toned physique in no time. You'll also calm your cravings, have a consistent source of energy, and won't feel fatigued throughout the day as you usually would.

The next step is to take the necessary action and put into practice what you have learnt. Don't forget to consult your doctor before you start any kind of diet, especially if you have some underlying condition.

www.ingramcontent.com/pod-product-compliance
Lightning Source LLC
Chambersburg PA
CBHW061232280526
45784CB00006B/2732